Vakare Rimkute

Adrenal Fatigue Relief Diet Cookbook: Revitalize Your Energy with Wholesome, Adrenal-Supportive Meals

Contents

1.

   1.

   2.

   3.

2.

   1.

   2.

3.

1.
2.
3.
4.
4.
    1.
    2.
    3.
    4.
5.
    1.
    2.
    3.
    4.
6.
    1.
    2.
    3.
    4.
7.
    1.
    2.
    3.
    4.
8.

1.

2.

3.

4.

9.

1.

2.

3.

4.

Chapter 1: Introduction

What is Adrenal Fatigue?

Adrenal fatigue is a term used to describe a collection of nonspecific symptoms, such as fatigue, body aches, and nervousness, which some people attribute to chronic stress and an overworking of the adrenal glands. The adrenal glands, located on top of each kidney, produce hormones, including cortisol, which plays a role in managing stress.

However, it's important to note that adrenal fatigue is not a medically recognized term or diagnosis in mainstream medicine. The concept is controversial, and there is limited scientific evidence to support the idea that chronic stress directly leads to a significant decline in adrenal function.

Importance of Diet in Adrenal Fatigue Relief:

1. **Nutrient Support:** A balanced and nutrient-rich diet provides essential vitamins and minerals that support adrenal function. Nutrients like vitamin C, B vitamins, magnesium, and zinc are crucial for adrenal health.

2. **Energy Balance:** Adrenal fatigue often leads to fatigue and low energy levels. A well-balanced diet helps maintain stable blood sugar levels, preventing energy crashes and supporting sustained energy throughout the day.

3. **Stress Reduction**: Certain foods and nutrients, such as omega-3 fatty acids and antioxidants, can help mitigate the impact of stress on the body. These components may have anti-inflammatory and calming effects.

4. **Avoidance of Trigger Foods**: Some foods, like caffeine, processed sugars, and excessive amounts of refined carbohydrates, can exacerbate adrenal fatigue symptoms. A carefully planned diet helps individuals avoid these triggers.

5. **Hormonal Balance:** Diet plays a role in hormonal balance, and imbalances can contribute to adrenal fatigue. For instance, a diet rich in fibre and healthy fats supports balanced hormone production.

6. **Gut Health**: The gut and adrenal function are interconnected. A diet that promotes a healthy gut microbiome can positively influence adrenal health. Probiotics and fibre-rich foods contribute to gut well-being.

7. **Hydration**: Proper hydration is vital for overall health, and it supports adrenal function. Dehydration can amplify stress on the body, so maintaining adequate fluid intake is crucial.

8. **Whole, Unprocessed Foods:** A diet focused on whole, unprocessed foods ensures a diverse range of nutrients. Processed foods often lack essential vitamins and minerals and may contribute to inflammation.

Key Nutrients for Adrenal Health:

1. **Vitamin C:**
   - Found in citrus fruits, strawberries, and bell peppers.
   - Supports adrenal gland function and helps in the production of stress hormones.

2. **B Vitamins:**
   - Sources include whole grains, leafy greens, and eggs.
   - Vital for energy production and stress response.

3. **Magnesium**:

   - Found in nuts, seeds, and leafy greens.

   - Helps regulate cortisol levels and supports overall adrenal function.

4. **Zinc**:

   - Sources include meat, seafood, and pumpkin seeds.

   - Important for immune function and helps modulate the stress response.

5. **Omega-3 Fatty Acids:**

   - Found in fatty fish, flaxseeds, and walnuts.

   - Anti-inflammatory and supports cognitive function during stress.

6. **Adaptogenic Herbs:**

   - Examples include ashwagandha, rhodiola, and holy basil.
   - Help the body adapt to stress and support adrenal function.

7. **Protein**:

   - Found in meat, fish, dairy, legumes.
   - Essential for tissue repair and supports overall energy levels.

8. **Iron**:

   - Sources include lean meats, beans, and lentils.

   - Important for preventing fatigue and supporting oxygen transport in the blood.

9. **Vitamin D:**

   - Obtained from sunlight, fatty fish, and fortified foods.

   - Plays a role in hormone regulation, including cortisol.

10. **Potassium**:

   - Found in bananas, potatoes, and leafy greens.

   - Balances sodium levels and supports overall adrenal health.

Chapter 2: Understanding Adrenal Fatigue

Symptoms and Signs:

1. Physical Symptoms:
- Fatigue and low energy levels
- Difficulty falling asleep or staying asleep
- Weight gain or difficulty losing weight
- Muscle weakness
- Digestive issues, such as bloating or constipation
- Changes in skin tone and appearance

2. Emotional Symptoms:
- Persistent feelings of tiredness or exhaustion
- Increased irritability or mood swings
- Difficulty handling stress
- Anxiety or depression
- Reduced ability to cope with everyday challenges

3. Behavioral Signs:
- Increased reliance on stimulants like caffeine
- Changes in appetite and food cravings
- Decreased libido
- Difficulty concentrating or experiencing brain fog

- Withdrawal from social activities

4. Circadian Rhythm Disruptions:

- Irregular sleep patterns

- Feeling more awake and alert in the evening

- Difficulty waking up in the morning

5. Impact on Daily Life:

- Challenges in maintaining a regular work schedule

- Impaired physical performance and exercise tolerance

- Strained relationships due to mood fluctuations

- Reduced overall quality of life

Causes and Triggers of Adrenal Fatigue:

1. **Chronic Stress:** Prolonged periods of stress, whether physical or emotional, can strain the adrenal glands, leading to fatigue. The chapter may discuss ways to identify and manage stressors.

2. **Poor Nutrition:** A diet lacking in essential nutrients can contribute to adrenal fatigue. The cookbook might emphasize the importance of a well-balanced diet to support adrenal health.

3. **Inadequate Sleep**: Insufficient or poor-quality sleep can impact adrenal function. The chapter could provide tips for improving sleep hygiene and establishing healthy sleep patterns.

4. **Overuse of Stimulants**: Excessive consumption of stimulants like caffeine and sugar can strain the adrenals. The cookbook might suggest alternatives and moderation in consumption.

5. **Lack of Physical Activity**: Sedentary lifestyles can contribute to adrenal fatigue. The chapter may encourage incorporating appropriate exercise to support overall well-being.

6. **Environmental Toxins:** Exposure to environmental pollutants and toxins can affect adrenal health. The cookbook might highlight ways to minimize exposure and support detoxification.

7. **Underlying Medical Conditions**: Certain health conditions, such as autoimmune disorders or chronic infections, can impact adrenal function. The chapter could provide insights into identifying and managing these conditions.

8. **Genetic Predisposition:** Some individuals may be genetically predisposed to adrenal issues. The cookbook may discuss how understanding genetic factors can guide personalized dietary and lifestyle choices.

9. **Imbalanced Blood Sugar Levels:** Fluctuations in blood sugar levels can stress the adrenals. The chapter might include guidance on maintaining stable blood sugar through proper nutrition.

9

10. **Hormonal Imbalances:** Imbalances in hormones, such as cortisol and thyroid hormones, can contribute to adrenal fatigue. The cookbook may offer dietary strategies to support hormonal balance.

Chapter 3: Breakfast Recipes

Energizing Smoothie Bowl:

Ingredients:

- 1 frozen banana

- 1 cup mixed berries (such as blueberries, strawberries, raspberries)

- 1/2 cup Greek yogurt

- 1/4 cup almond milk (adjust for desired consistency)

- 1 tablespoon chia seeds

- 1 tablespoon honey or maple syrup (optional, for sweetness)

- Toppings: sliced kiwi, granola, pumpkin seeds, shredded coconut

Instructions:

1. **Blend the Base:**

- In a blender, combine the frozen banana, mixed berries, Greek yoghurt, almond milk, and chia seeds.

- Blend until smooth and creamy. Add more almond milk if needed to achieve your preferred consistency.

2. **Taste and Sweeten (Optional):**

   - Taste the smoothie mixture and add honey or maple syrup if you desire extra sweetness. Blend again to combine.

3. **Prepare the Bowl:**

   - Pour the smoothie into a bowl.

4. **Add Toppings:**

   - Decorate the smoothie bowl with sliced kiwi, granola, pumpkin seeds, and shredded coconut.

5. **Customize**:

   - Feel free to get creative with additional toppings like fresh berries, nuts, or a drizzle of nut butter.

6. **Serve and Enjoy:**

   - Grab a spoon and enjoy your energizing smoothie bowl!

Quinoa Porridge with Berries:

Ingredients:

   - 1/2 cup quinoa, rinsed

   - 1 cup almond milk (or any preferred milk)

   - 1/2 teaspoon vanilla extract

   - 1 tablespoon maple syrup or honey (adjust to taste)

- A pinch of salt

- 1/2 cup mixed berries (strawberries, blueberries, raspberries)

- 1 tablespoon chopped nuts (e.g., almonds, walnuts)

- Optional toppings: Greek yoghurt, additional berries, a drizzle of honey

Instructions:

1. **Rinse the Quinoa**:

Rinse quinoa under cold water to remove any bitterness.

2. **Cook Quinoa:**

In a medium saucepan, combine rinsed quinoa, almond milk, vanilla extract, and a pinch of salt. Bring to a boil, then reduce heat to low, cover, and simmer for about 15-20 minutes or until quinoa is cooked and has absorbed most of the liquid.

3. **Sweeten the Porridge:**

Stir in maple syrup or honey to sweeten the porridge. Adjust the sweetness according to your taste preference.

4. **Prepare Berries**:

While the quinoa is cooking, wash and slice the berries.

5. **Assemble the Porridge**:

Once the quinoa is ready, spoon it into bowls. Top with mixed berries and chopped nuts.

6. **Optional Toppings:**

Add a dollop of Greek yoghurt, extra berries, and a drizzle of honey if desired.

7. **Serve**:

Serve warm and enjoy your nutritious and delicious Quinoa Porridge with Berries!

Avocado and Egg Breakfast Wrap:

Ingredients:

- 1 large avocado, mashed
- 2 large eggs
- Salt and pepper to taste
- 2 whole-grain or gluten-free wraps
- 1/2 cup cherry tomatoes, sliced
- 1/4 cup red onion, finely chopped
- Fresh cilantro, chopped (optional)

Instructions:

1. **Prepare the Avocado Mash**:

- Cut the avocado in half, remove the pit, and scoop out the flesh into a bowl.

- Mash the avocado using a fork until smooth.

- Season with salt and pepper to taste.

2. **Cook the Eggs:**

- In a non-stick skillet over medium heat, crack the eggs and cook to your desired doneness (scrambled, fried, or poached).

- Season the eggs with salt and pepper.

3. **Warm the Wraps:**

- Heat the wraps in a dry skillet for about 10-15 seconds on each side or as per package instructions.

4. **Assemble the Breakfast Wrap:**

- Lay out the warmed wraps on a flat surface.

- Spread a generous portion of the mashed avocado onto each wrap, leaving some space around the edges.

5. **Add Eggs and Toppings:**

- Place the cooked eggs on top of the mashed avocado.

- Sprinkle sliced cherry tomatoes and finely chopped red onion over the eggs.

6. **Optional Garnish:**

- Add a sprinkle of fresh cilantro for added flavour and freshness.

7. **Fold and Serve:**

- Carefully fold the sides of the wrap over the filling to create a burrito-style wrap.

- Serve immediately and enjoy your nutritious Avocado and Egg Breakfast Wrap!

Chia Seed Pudding with Nuts and Seeds:

Ingredients:

- 1/4 cup chia seeds
    - 1 cup almond milk (or any milk of your choice)
    - 1-2 tablespoons maple syrup or honey (adjust to taste)
    - 1/2 teaspoon vanilla extract
    - A pinch of salt
    - 2 tablespoons chopped nuts (e.g., almonds, walnuts)
    - 1 tablespoon mixed seeds (e.g., chia seeds, flaxseeds, pumpkin seeds)

Instructions:

1. **Mix Chia Seeds and Liquid**:
In a bowl, combine chia seeds, almond milk, maple syrup or honey, vanilla extract, and a pinch of salt. Stir well to ensure the chia seeds are evenly distributed.

2. **Let it Sit:**

Cover the bowl and refrigerate for at least 2-3 hours, or ideally overnight. This allows the chia seeds to absorb the liquid and create a pudding-like consistency.

3. **Stir Again:**

After the initial setting time, give the mixture a good stir. This helps prevent clumps and ensures a smoother texture.

4. **Add Nuts and Seeds:**

Mix in the chopped nuts and seeds of your choice. This adds a delightful crunch and boosts the nutritional content of the pudding.

5. **Adjust Sweetness:**

Taste the pudding and adjust sweetness if needed by adding more maple syrup or honey. Stir well to incorporate any additional sweetener.

6. **Serve:**

Spoon the chia seed pudding into individual serving bowls or jars. You can layer it with additional nuts and seeds for presentation.

7. **Optional Toppings:**

Garnish with extra nuts, seeds, or a drizzle of honey before serving. Fresh berries or sliced fruit also make excellent toppings.

Chapter 4: Lunch Recipes

Kale and Chickpea Salad with Lemon-Tahini Dressing:

Ingredients:

For the Salad:
- 4 cups chopped kale, stems removed
- 1 can (15 oz) chickpeas, drained and rinsed
- 1 cup cherry tomatoes, halved
- 1 cucumber, diced
- 1/4 cup red onion, finely chopped
- 1/3 cup crumbled feta cheese (optional)
- 1/4 cup chopped fresh parsley (optional)

For the Lemon-Tahini Dressing:
- 3 tablespoons tahini
- 2 tablespoons olive oil
- 2 tablespoons fresh lemon juice
- 1 garlic clove, minced
- 1 teaspoon honey or maple syrup
- Salt and pepper to taste
- Water (as needed to adjust consistency)

Instructions:

1. **Prepare the Salad:**
   - In a large bowl, massage the chopped kale with a bit of olive oil for a few minutes to soften it.

2. **Add the Vegetables:**
   - Add chickpeas, cherry tomatoes, cucumber, red onion, and any optional ingredients (feta cheese, parsley) to the bowl with kale.

3. **Make the Dressing**:
   - In a separate small bowl, whisk together tahini, olive oil, fresh lemon juice, minced garlic, honey or maple syrup, salt, and pepper.

4. **Combine Salad and Dressing**:
   - Pour the lemon-tahini dressing over the salad.

5. **Toss Well:**
   - Toss the salad thoroughly, ensuring the dressing coats all the ingredients evenly.

6. **Adjust Consistency:**
   - If the dressing is too thick, you can add a little water, one tablespoon at a time, until you reach your desired consistency.

7. **Serve**:

- Plate the salad and serve immediately. Optionally, garnish with additional parsley or a sprinkle of feta cheese.

8. **Enjoy**:

- Enjoy your nutritious and flavorful Kale and Chickpea Salad!

Turkey and Vegetable Lettuce Wraps:

Ingredients:

- 1 lb ground turkey
    - 1 tablespoon olive oil
    - 1 small onion, finely chopped
    - 2 cloves garlic, minced
    - 1 red bell pepper, diced
    - 1 zucchini, diced
    - 1 carrot, julienned
    - 2 tablespoons soy sauce (or tamari for a gluten-free option)
    - 1 tablespoon hoisin sauce
    - 1 teaspoon sesame oil
    - 1 teaspoon fresh ginger, grated
    - Salt and pepper, to taste
    - Butter or iceberg lettuce leaves for wrapping

Instructions:

1. **Cooking the Turkey:**
   - Heat olive oil in a large skillet over medium heat.
   - Add chopped onion and garlic, sautéing until fragrant.
   - Add ground turkey, breaking it up with a spatula. Cook until browned and cooked through.

2. **Adding Vegetables:**
   - Stir in diced bell pepper, zucchini, and julienned carrot. Cook for a few minutes until vegetables are tender-crisp.

3. **Seasoning**:
   - In a small bowl, mix soy sauce, hoisin sauce, sesame oil, and grated ginger.
   - Pour the sauce over the turkey and vegetable mixture. Stir well to coat evenly.
   - Season with salt and pepper to taste.

4. **Assembling Wraps:**
   - Spoon the turkey and vegetable mixture onto individual lettuce leaves.
   - Optionally, drizzle with extra soy sauce or hoisin sauce for added flavour.

5. **Serve**:
   - Arrange the lettuce wraps on a serving platter.

- Serve immediately and enjoy the flavorful and nutritious Turkey and Vegetable Lettuce Wraps!

Sweet Potato and Lentil Soup:

Ingredients:

- 1 tablespoon olive oil
- 1 onion, diced
- 2 garlic cloves, minced
- 1 teaspoon ground cumin
- 1 teaspoon ground coriander
- 1/2 teaspoon ground turmeric
- 1/2 teaspoon smoked paprika
- 1 large sweet potato, peeled and diced
- 1 cup red lentils, rinsed and drained
- 6 cups vegetable broth
- Salt and pepper to taste
- Fresh cilantro or parsley for garnish (optional)

Instructions:

1. Heat the olive oil in a large pot over medium heat. Add the diced onion and sauté until softened.

2. Add the minced garlic and sauté for an additional minute until fragrant.

3. Stir in the ground cumin, ground coriander, ground turmeric, and smoked paprika. Cook for another minute to toast the spices.

4. Add the diced sweet potato and red lentils to the pot. Stir well to coat them in the spices.

5. Pour in the vegetable broth and bring the soup to a boil. Once boiling, reduce the heat to low, cover the pot, and let it simmer for about 20-25 minutes or until the sweet potatoes and lentils are tender.

6. Use an immersion blender to blend the soup until smooth. If you don't have an immersion blender, carefully transfer the soup in batches to a blender and blend until smooth. Be cautious when blending hot liquids.

7. Season the soup with salt and pepper to taste. Adjust the seasoning as needed.

8. Ladle the soup into bowls, and if desired, garnish with fresh cilantro or parsley.

Grilled Salmon with Quinoa and Steamed Vegetables:

Grilled salmon:

Ingredients:

- 4 salmon fillets

- 2 tablespoons olive oil

- 2 cloves garlic, minced

- 1 teaspoon lemon zest

- 2 tablespoons lemon juice

- 1 teaspoon dried oregano

- Salt and pepper to taste

Instructions:

1. Preheat the grill to medium-high heat.

2. In a small bowl, mix olive oil, minced garlic, lemon zest, lemon juice, dried oregano, salt, and pepper to create a marinade.

3. Place salmon fillets in a shallow dish and brush both sides with the marinade. Let it marinate for at least 15 minutes.

4. Grill the salmon for about 4-5 minutes per side or until the salmon is cooked through and easily flakes with a fork.

Quinoa:

Ingredients:

- 1 cup quinoa

- 2 cups water or vegetable broth

- 1/2 teaspoon salt

Instructions:

1. Rinse the quinoa under cold water.

2. In a medium saucepan, combine quinoa, water or broth, and salt.

3. Bring to a boil, then reduce heat to low, cover, and simmer for 15 minutes, or until the quinoa is cooked and liquid is absorbed.

4. Fluff the quinoa with a fork.

Steamed Vegetables:

Ingredients:

- Assorted vegetables (broccoli, carrots, snap peas, etc.), washed and chopped

- 1 tablespoon olive oil

- Salt and pepper to taste

Instructions:

1. Fill a steamer basket with the chopped vegetables.

2. Bring water to a boil in the steamer pot.

3. Place the steamer basket over the boiling water, cover, and steam for about 5-7 minutes or until vegetables are tender but still crisp.

4. Drizzle olive oil over the steamed vegetables and season with salt and pepper.

Assembling the Dish:

1. Place a serving of quinoa on each plate.

2. Top the quinoa with grilled salmon fillets.

3. Arrange the steamed vegetables on the side.

4. Garnish with fresh herbs or a wedge of lemon if desired.

Chapter 5: Snack Recipes

Energy-Boosting Trail Mix:

Ingredients:

1. 1 cup almonds, raw or lightly toasted
2. 1 cup walnuts
3. 1/2 cup pumpkin seeds
4. 1/2 cup sunflower seeds
5. 1/2 cup dried cranberries
6. 1/2 cup unsweetened coconut flakes
7. 1/2 cup dark chocolate chips (70% cocoa or higher)
8. 1 teaspoon cinnamon
9. 1/2 teaspoon sea salt

Instructions:

1. If the almonds are raw, you can lightly toast them in a dry skillet over medium heat for a few minutes until they become fragrant. Let them cool.

2. In a large mixing bowl, combine almonds, walnuts, pumpkin seeds, sunflower seeds, dried cranberries, coconut flakes, and dark chocolate chips.

3. Sprinkle cinnamon and sea salt over the mixture.

4. Toss all the ingredients together until well combined. Make sure the cinnamon and salt are evenly distributed.

5. Store the trail mix in an airtight container or portion it into smaller snack-sized bags for convenient grab-and-go servings.

Optional Additions:
- Chia seeds or flaxseeds for added omega-3 fatty acids.
- Dried apricots or raisins for natural sweetness.
- Your favourite nuts or seeds based on personal preference.

Greek Yogurt Parfait with Fresh Fruit:

Ingredients:
- 1 cup Greek yogurt
- 2 tablespoons honey or maple syrup (adjust to taste)
- 1 teaspoon vanilla extract
- 1 cup mixed fresh fruits (berries, sliced kiwi, banana, etc.)
- 1/4 cup granola
- 2 tablespoons chopped nuts (e.g., almonds, walnuts)

Instructions:

1. **Prepare Greek Yogurt Mixture**:

   - In a bowl, combine Greek yoghurt, honey or maple syrup, and vanilla extract.

   - Mix well until the sweetener is evenly distributed.

2. **Layering the Parfait:**

   - In a glass or a bowl, start by adding a layer of the Greek yoghurt mixture at the bottom.

3. **Add Fresh Fruits:**

   - Add a layer of mixed fresh fruits on top of the yoghurt mixture. Use a variety of fruits for a colourful and flavorful parfait.

4. **Sprinkle Granola:**

   - Sprinkle a layer of granola over the fresh fruits. This adds a delightful crunch to the parfait.

5. **Repeat Layers:**

   - Repeat the layers by adding more Greek yoghurt, fresh fruits, and granola until you reach the top of the glass or bowl.

6. **Top with Nuts:**

   - Finish off the parfait by sprinkling chopped nuts on the top layer. This adds an extra layer of texture and healthy fats.

7. **Drizzle with Honey (Optional)**:

   - For an extra touch of sweetness, you can drizzle a bit more honey or maple syrup on the top.

8. **Serve and Enjoy:**

- Serve the Greek Yogurt Parfait immediately and enjoy a delicious and nutritious treat!

Roasted Chickpeas with Spices:

Ingredients:

- 2 cans (15 ounces each) chickpeas, drained and rinsed
- 2 tablespoons olive oil
- 1 teaspoon ground cumin
- 1 teaspoon smoked paprika
- 1/2 teaspoon garlic powder
- 1/2 teaspoon onion powder
- 1/4 teaspoon cayenne pepper (adjust to taste)
- Salt and black pepper to taste

Instructions:

1. **Preheat the Oven:** Preheat your oven to 400°F (200°C).

2. **Prepare Chickpeas**: Rinse and drain the chickpeas thoroughly. Pat them dry with a clean kitchen towel or paper towel. Removing excess moisture helps them get crispy.

3. **Seasoning Mixture**: In a bowl, mix olive oil, ground cumin, smoked paprika, garlic powder, onion powder, cayenne pepper, salt, and black pepper. Adjust the spice levels according to your preference.

4. **Coat Chickpeas**: Add the dried chickpeas to the seasoning mixture and toss until they are well coated.

5. **Spread on Baking Sheet**: Spread the seasoned chickpeas in a single layer on a baking sheet. Make sure they are evenly distributed.

6. **Roast in the Oven:** Place the baking sheet in the preheated oven and roast for about 25-30 minutes or until the chickpeas are golden brown and crispy. Shake the baking sheet or stir the chickpeas halfway through the roasting time for even crispiness.

7. **Cool and Enjoy**: Once roasted, remove the chickpeas from the oven and let them cool for a few minutes. They will continue to crisp up as they cool.

8. **Serve**: Enjoy the roasted chickpeas as a snack or as a crunchy topping for salads and soups.

Nut Butter and Banana Slices:

Ingredients:

- 1 banana, sliced
- 2 tablespoons nut butter (almond, peanut, or your choice)
- Optional toppings: chia seeds, honey, or a sprinkle of cinnamon

Instructions:

1. **Slice the Banana**: Peel the banana and cut it into thin slices. Arrange the slices on a plate or cutting board.

2. **Spread Nut Butter**: Take your preferred nut butter and spread it onto each banana slice. You can use the back of a spoon or a butter knife for this.

3. **Optional Toppings**: Sprinkle chia seeds, drizzle honey, or add a pinch of cinnamon for extra flavour and nutritional benefits.

4. **Serve**: Your Nut Butter and Banana Slices are ready to be enjoyed! Arrange them on a plate and savour this quick and healthy snack.

Chapter 6: Dinner Recipes

Baked Chicken with Garlic and Herbs:

Ingredients:

- 4 boneless, skinless chicken breasts

- 4 cloves of garlic, minced

- 2 tablespoons olive oil

- 1 teaspoon dried oregano

- 1 teaspoon dried thyme

- 1 teaspoon dried rosemary

- Salt and pepper to taste

- 1 lemon, sliced (optional for garnish)

Instructions:

1. Preheat your oven to 400°F (200°C).

2. In a small bowl, mix minced garlic, olive oil, dried oregano, dried thyme, dried rosemary, salt, and pepper. This creates the herb marinade.

3. Place the chicken breasts in a baking dish. Using a brush or your hands, coat each chicken breast with the herb marinade, ensuring they are well-covered.

4. If you have time, let the chicken marinate for about 15-30 minutes to enhance the flavours. If you're short on time, you can proceed to the next step.

5. Place the baking dish in the preheated oven and bake for approximately 20-25 minutes or until the chicken reaches an internal temperature of 165°F (74°C).

6. If desired, you can broil the chicken for an additional 2-3 minutes at the end to achieve a golden-brown finish.

7. Once cooked, remove the baking dish from the oven, and let the chicken rest for a few minutes before serving.

8. Garnish with fresh herbs or lemon slices if desired.

Serve the baked chicken with your favourite side dishes, such as roasted vegetables, quinoa, or a fresh salad.

Stir-fried tofu with Broccoli and Bell Peppers:

Ingredients:

- 1 block of firm tofu, pressed and cubed
    - 2 cups broccoli florets
    - 1 red bell pepper, thinly sliced
    - 1 yellow bell pepper, thinly sliced
    - 3 cloves garlic, minced
    - 1 tablespoon ginger, grated
    - 3 tablespoons soy sauce (or tamari for a gluten-free option)
    - 2 tablespoons sesame oil
    - 1 tablespoon rice vinegar
    - 1 tablespoon cornstarch mixed with 2 tablespoons water (optional, for thickening)
    - 2 green onions, sliced (for garnish)
    - Sesame seeds (for garnish)
    - Cooked brown rice or quinoa (for serving)

Instructions:

1. **Prepare Tofu:**
    - Press the tofu to remove excess water. Cut it into cubes.

2. **Stir-Fry Tofu**:
    - Heat 1 tablespoon of sesame oil in a large skillet or wok over medium-high heat.

- Add the tofu cubes and cook until they are golden brown on all sides. Remove tofu from the pan and set aside.

3. **Vegetable Stir-Fry**:
- In the same pan, add another tablespoon of sesame oil.
- Add minced garlic and grated ginger, and sauté for about 1 minute until fragrant.
- Add broccoli and bell peppers. Stir-fry for 3-4 minutes until the vegetables are slightly tender but still vibrant.

4. **Combine Tofu and Vegetables**:
- Return the cooked tofu to the pan with the vegetables.

5. **Sauce**:
- In a small bowl, mix soy sauce and rice vinegar. Pour the sauce over the tofu and vegetables. Toss everything to coat evenly.

6. **Optional Thickening:**
- If you prefer a thicker sauce, mix cornstarch with water to create a slurry. Stir it into the pan and cook until the sauce thickens.

7. **Garnish and Serve:**
- Garnish with sliced green onions and sesame seeds.
- Serve the stir-fry over cooked brown rice or quinoa.

Zucchini Noodles with Pesto and Cherry Tomatoes:

Ingredients:
- 4 medium-sized zucchini, spiralized into noodles
- 1 cup cherry tomatoes, halved
- 1/2 cup fresh basil leaves, packed
- 1/4 cup pine nuts
- 1/2 cup grated Parmesan cheese
- 2 cloves garlic, minced
- 1/2 cup extra-virgin olive oil
- Salt and pepper to taste

Instructions:

1. **Make the Pesto**:
   - In a food processor, combine the basil, pine nuts, Parmesan cheese, and minced garlic.
   - Pulse until the ingredients are finely chopped.
   - With the food processor running, gradually add the olive oil in a steady stream until the pesto reaches a smooth consistency.
   - Season with salt and pepper to taste. Set aside.

2. **Prepare the Zucchini Noodles**:
   - Spiralize the zucchini into noodles using a spiralizer.
   - If you don't have a spiralizer, you can use a vegetable peeler to create thin ribbons.

3. **Cook the Zucchini Noodles:**

   - Heat a large skillet over medium heat.

   - Add a bit of olive oil to the skillet.

   - Sauté the zucchini noodles for 2-3 minutes, just until they are slightly softened but still have a bit of crunch.

4. **Combine with Pesto and Cherry Tomatoes:**

   - Add the cherry tomato halves to the skillet with the zucchini noodles.

   - Pour the prepared pesto over the noodles and tomatoes.

   - Gently toss everything together until the zucchini noodles are well coated with pesto and the cherry tomatoes are evenly distributed.

5. **Serve:**

   - Transfer the zucchini noodles, pesto, and cherry tomatoes to serving plates.

   - Optionally, garnish with additional grated Parmesan cheese and fresh basil leaves.

Lentil and Vegetable Stew:

Ingredients:

- 1 cup dried brown or green lentils, rinsed and drained
- 1 onion, finely chopped
- 2 carrots, diced
- 2 celery stalks, chopped
- 3 cloves garlic, minced
- 1 can (14 oz) diced tomatoes
- 1 zucchini, diced
- 1 red bell pepper, diced
- 4 cups vegetable broth
- 1 teaspoon ground cumin
- 1 teaspoon smoked paprika
- 1/2 teaspoon turmeric
- Salt and pepper to taste
- 2 tablespoons olive oil
- Fresh parsley for garnish

Instructions:

1. **Prepare Lentils**: Rinse lentils under cold water and set aside.

2. **Sauté Vegetables**: In a large pot, heat olive oil over medium heat. Add onions, carrots, and celery. Sauté until vegetables are softened, about 5 minutes.

3. **Add Aromatics**: Add minced garlic, cumin, smoked paprika, and turmeric. Sauté for an additional 1-2 minutes until fragrant.

4. **Combine Ingredients**: Stir in lentils, diced tomatoes, zucchini, red bell pepper, and vegetable broth. Bring the mixture to a boil.

5. **Simmer**: Reduce heat to low, cover the pot, and let it simmer for about 25-30 minutes or until lentils are tender.

6. **Season**: Season the stew with salt and pepper to taste. Adjust the seasoning if needed.

7. **Serve**: Ladle the stew into bowls, garnish with fresh parsley, and serve   hot.

Chapter 7: Side Dishes

Roasted Brussels Sprouts with Balsamic Glaze:

Ingredients:

- 1 lb Brussels sprouts, trimmed and halved
- 2 tablespoons olive oil
- Salt and pepper to taste
- 2 tablespoons balsamic glaze (store-bought or homemade)

Instructions:

1. **Preheat the Oven:**

   - Preheat your oven to 400°F (200°C).

2. **Prepare Brussels Sprouts:**

   - Trim the ends of the Brussels sprouts and cut them in half. Remove any loose or yellowed outer leaves.

3. **Coat with Olive Oil:**

   - Place the halved Brussels sprouts in a mixing bowl. Drizzle olive oil over them, ensuring they are evenly coated. Toss them to coat evenly.

4. **Season with Salt and Pepper:**

- Season the Brussels sprouts with salt and pepper according to your taste. Toss them again to distribute the seasonings.

5. **Roast in the Oven:**

- Spread the Brussels sprouts in a single layer on a baking sheet. Roast in the preheated oven for about 20-25 minutes or until they are golden brown and crispy on the edges. Toss halfway through the roasting time for even cooking.

6. **Drizzle with Balsamic Glaze:**

- Once the Brussels sprouts are roasted to your liking, remove them from the oven. Drizzle the balsamic glaze over the roasted sprouts while they are still hot.

7. **Serve:**

- Transfer the Brussels sprouts to a serving dish and serve immediately. The balsamic glaze adds a sweet and tangy flavour that complements the nutty taste of the roasted Brussels sprouts.

Quinoa Pilaf with Mixed Vegetables:

Ingredients:

- 1 cup quinoa, rinsed and drained

- 2 cups vegetable broth or water

- 1 tablespoon olive oil

- 1 small onion, finely chopped

- 2 cloves garlic, minced

- 1 carrot, diced

- 1 bell pepper (any colour), diced

- 1 zucchini, diced

- 1 cup cherry tomatoes, halved

- 1 teaspoon dried oregano

- Salt and pepper to taste

- Fresh parsley, chopped (for garnish)

Instructions:

1. **Rinse the Quinoa:**

   - Rinse the quinoa under cold water to remove any bitterness.

2. **Cook the Quinoa:**

   - In a medium saucepan, combine the quinoa and vegetable broth (or water).

   - Bring to a boil, then reduce heat to low, cover, and simmer for about 15 minutes or until the quinoa is cooked and the liquid is absorbed.

   - Remove from heat and let it sit covered for 5 minutes. Fluff the quinoa with a fork.

3. **Sauté Vegetables:**

   - In a large skillet, heat olive oil over medium heat.

- Add chopped onion and garlic, and sauté until softened and fragrant.

4. **Add Vegetables:**

- Add diced carrot, bell pepper, and zucchini to the skillet. Sauté for about 5-7 minutes until the vegetables are tender but still crisp.

5. **Combine Quinoa and Vegetables:**

- Add the cooked quinoa to the skillet with sautéed vegetables.
- Gently stir to combine, allowing the flavours to meld.

6. **Season and Garnish:**

- Season the pilaf with dried oregano, salt, and pepper to taste.
- Toss in halved cherry tomatoes and cook for an additional 2-3 minutes until they soften slightly.
- Garnish with freshly chopped parsley.

7. **Serve:**

- Spoon the quinoa pilaf onto serving plates or into a large bowl.

Mashed Cauliflower with Garlic:

Ingredients:

- 1 large head of cauliflower, washed and cut into florets

- 4 cloves of garlic, minced

- 2 tablespoons olive oil

- Salt and pepper to taste

- Fresh chives or parsley for garnish (optional)

Instructions:

1. **Steam the Cauliflower**:

- Place the cauliflower florets in a steamer basket over a pot of boiling water.

- Steam for about 10-15 minutes or until the cauliflower is tender and easily pierced with a fork.

2. **Sauté Garlic**:

- While the cauliflower is steaming, heat olive oil in a pan over medium heat.

- Add minced garlic and sauté for 1-2 minutes until fragrant. Be careful not to burn the garlic.

3. **Mash the Cauliflower:**

- Once the cauliflower is tender, transfer it to a large bowl.

- Use a potato masher or an immersion blender to mash the cauliflower until smooth. You can also use a food processor for a creamier texture.

4. **Combine with Garlic:**

- Add the sautéed garlic and olive oil to the mashed cauliflower.

- Season with salt and pepper to taste.

5. **Blend Well:**

   - Mix everything well, ensuring that the garlic is evenly distributed.

6. **Garnish (Optional):**

   - Garnish with fresh chives or parsley for added flavour and a pop of colour.

7. **Serve Warm**:

   - Serve the mashed cauliflower warm as a delicious and nutritious alternative to traditional mashed potatoes.

Steamed Asparagus with Lemon:

Ingredients:

   - 1 bunch of fresh asparagus, trimmed
   - 1 lemon, thinly sliced
   - 2 tablespoons olive oil
   - Salt and pepper to taste
   - Fresh parsley for garnish (optional)

Instructions:

1. **Prepare Asparagus**:

   - Wash the asparagus under cold water and trim off the tough ends.

2. **Steam Asparagus**:

   - Place a steamer basket in a pot with a small amount of water, ensuring the water doesn't touch the bottom of the basket.

   - Add the trimmed asparagus to the steamer basket.

3. **Steam**:

   - Cover the pot and steam the asparagus for about 3-5 minutes, or until they are bright green and tender-crisp. Avoid overcooking, as you want the asparagus to retain some crunch.

4. **Lemon Slices:**

   - While the asparagus is steaming, heat olive oil in a small pan over medium heat. Add lemon slices and sauté briefly until they're slightly caramelized.

5. **Combine**:

   - Once the asparagus is steamed, transfer it to a serving platter. Drizzle the sautéed lemon slices and oil over the asparagus.

6. **Season**:

   - Season with salt and pepper to taste. Toss gently to coat the asparagus evenly.

7. **Garnish**:

- If desired, garnish with fresh parsley for added flavour and presentation.

47

8. **Serve**:

- Serve the steamed asparagus with lemon slices immediately, either as a side dish or a light appetizer.

Chapter 8: Dessert Recipes

Berry and Coconut Bliss Balls:

Ingredients:

- 1 cup mixed berries (strawberries, blueberries, raspberries)
- 1 cup shredded coconut (plus extra for coating)
- 1 cup rolled oats
- 1/2 cup almond butter
- 1/4 cup honey or maple syrup
- 1 teaspoon vanilla extract
- Pinch of salt

instructions:

1. **Prepare Berries**: If using fresh berries, wash and pat them dry. If using frozen berries, make sure to thaw and drain any excess liquid.

2. **Blend Ingredients**: In a food processor, combine the mixed berries, shredded coconut, rolled oats, almond butter, honey or maple syrup, vanilla extract, and a pinch of salt. Blend until the mixture forms a sticky dough.

3. **Shape into Balls:** Scoop out small portions of the mixture and roll them between your palms to form bite-sized balls.

4. **Coat with Coconut:** Roll each bliss ball in additional shredded coconut to coat the exterior.

5. **Chill:** Place the bliss balls on a tray or plate and refrigerate for at least 30 minutes to firm up.

6. **Serve:** Once chilled, your Berry and Coconut Bliss Balls are ready to be served. Enjoy them as a healthy snack or dessert!

Dark Chocolate Avocado Mousse:

Ingredients:

- 2 ripe avocados

- 1/4 cup unsweetened cocoa powder

- 1/4 cup dark chocolate chips (at least 70% cocoa)

- 1/4 cup maple syrup or honey

- 1 teaspoon vanilla extract

- A pinch of salt

- Optional toppings: shaved dark chocolate, fresh berries, or chopped nuts

Instructions:

1. **Melt the Dark Chocolate:**

   - In a heatproof bowl, melt the dark chocolate chips. You can do this by placing the bowl over a pot of simmering water (double boiler) or by melting it in short bursts in the microwave. Stir until smooth and set aside to cool slightly.

2. **Prepare the Avocados:**

   - Cut the avocados in half, remove the pits, and scoop the flesh into a blender or food processor.

3. **Blend Ingredients:**

   - Add the melted dark chocolate, cocoa powder, maple syrup or honey, vanilla extract, and a pinch of salt to the blender or food processor.

4. **Blend Until Smooth:**

   - Blend all the ingredients until you achieve a smooth and creamy consistency. Scrape down the sides of the blender or food processor as needed.

5. **Taste and Adjust:**

   - Taste the mousse and adjust the sweetness if necessary by adding more maple syrup or honey.

6. Chill:

- Transfer the mousse to serving bowls or glasses and refrigerate for at least 30 minutes to allow it to set.

7. Serve:

- Once chilled, garnish with shaved dark chocolate, fresh berries, or chopped nuts before serving.

Baked Apples with Cinnamon and Walnuts:

Ingredients:

- 4 large apples (such as Honeycrisp or Granny Smith)
- 1/4 cup chopped walnuts
- 2 tablespoons maple syrup or honey
- 1 teaspoon ground cinnamon
- 1 tablespoon melted coconut oil or butter
- A pinch of salt

Instructions:

1. **Preheat the Oven:**

- Preheat your oven to 375°F (190°C).

2. **Prepare Apples:**

   - Wash and core the apples, leaving the bottom intact to create a well for the filling.

3. **Make the Filling:**

   - In a bowl, combine chopped walnuts, maple syrup or honey, ground cinnamon, melted coconut oil or butter, and a pinch of salt. Mix well.

4. **Fill the Apples:**

   - Stuff each cored apple with the walnut mixture, pressing it down slightly.

5. **Bake:**

   - Place the filled apples in a baking dish.
   - Bake in the preheated oven for 25-30 minutes or until the apples are tender.

6. **Baste Occasionally:**

   - Optionally, you can baste the apples with the juices from the baking dish halfway through to keep them moist.

7. **Serve Warm:**

   - Once baked, remove from the oven and let them cool slightly.
   - Serve the baked apples warm, and you can drizzle any remaining juices from the baking dish over the top.

Almond Flour Banana Bread:

Ingredients:
- 3 ripe bananas, mashed
- 3 large eggs
- 1/4 cup coconut oil, melted
- 1/4 cup honey or maple syrup
- 1 teaspoon vanilla extract
- 2 1/2 cups almond flour
- 1/2 teaspoon baking soda
- 1/2 teaspoon baking powder
- 1/4 teaspoon salt
- 1 teaspoon ground cinnamon (optional)
- 1/2 cup chopped nuts or chocolate chips (optional)

Instructions:

1. Preheat your oven to 350°F (175°C). Grease a loaf pan or line it with parchment paper.

2. In a large mixing bowl, combine the mashed bananas, eggs, melted coconut oil, honey or maple syrup, and vanilla extract. Mix well until the ingredients are thoroughly combined.

3. In a separate bowl, whisk together the almond flour, baking soda, baking powder, salt, and cinnamon if using.

4. Gradually add the dry ingredients to the wet ingredients, stirring until just combined. Be careful not to overmix.

5. If desired, fold in chopped nuts or chocolate chips into the batter.

6. Pour the batter into the prepared loaf pan, spreading it evenly.

7. Bake in the preheated oven for 50-60 minutes or until a toothpick inserted into the centre comes out clean.

8. Allow the banana bread to cool in the pan for about 10 minutes, then transfer it to a wire rack to cool completely before slicing.

9. Slice and enjoy the delicious and moist almond flour banana bread!

Chapter 9: Beverages

Herbal Teas for Adrenal Support:

1. Adaptogenic Blend Tea:

   - Ingredients:

   - 1 teaspoon ashwagandha root

   - 1 teaspoon rhodiola root

   - 1 teaspoon licorice root

- Instructions:

   - Steep the herbs in hot water for 10-15 minutes.

   - Strain and enjoy. Add honey or lemon if desired.

2. Holy Basil (Tulsi) Tea:

   - Ingredients:

   - 1 tablespoon dried holy basil leaves or 2-3 fresh leaves

   - 1 cup hot water

- Instructions:

   - Place the holy basil leaves in a cup.

   - Pour hot water over the leaves and steep for 5-7 minutes.

   - Strain and sip slowly.

3. Nettle and Peppermint Tea:

- **Ingredients:**
- 1 tablespoon dried nettle leaves
- 1 teaspoon dried peppermint leaves
- 1 cup hot water

- Instructions:
- Combine nettle and peppermint leaves in a cup.
- Pour hot water over the leaves and steep for 10 minutes.
- Strain before drinking.

4. Licorice Root Tea:

- **Ingredients:**
- 1 teaspoon dried licorice root
- 1 cup hot water

- Instructions:
- Place the liquorice root in a cup.
- Pour hot water over the root and steep for 5-10 minutes.
- Strain and enjoy.

5. Ginger and Lemon Balm Tea:

- **Ingredients:**
- 1 tablespoon fresh ginger slices
- 1 tablespoon dried lemon balm leaves
- 1 cup hot water

- Instructions:

- Combine ginger and lemon balm in a cup.

- Pour hot water over the herbs and steep for 7-10 minutes.

- Strain before drinking.

6. **Chamomile and Lavender Tea:**

- Ingredients:

- 1 tablespoon dried chamomile flowers

- 1 teaspoon dried lavender buds

- 1 cup hot water

- Instructions:

- Mix chamomile and lavender in a cup.

- Pour hot water over the herbs and steep for 5-7 minutes.

- Strain and enjoy before bedtime.

Green Smoothie for Energy:

Ingredients:

1. 1 cup fresh spinach leaves

2. 1/2 cucumber, peeled and sliced

3. 1/2 green apple, cored and chopped

4. 1/2 banana

5. 1/2 lemon, juiced

6. 1 tablespoon chia seeds

7. 1 cup coconut water or almond milk

8. Ice cubes (optional)

Instructions:

1. Place the fresh spinach leaves, cucumber slices, chopped green apple, banana, and chia seeds in a blender.

2. Squeeze the juice of half a lemon into the blender.

3. Pour in the coconut water or almond milk.

4. If desired, add a handful of ice cubes for a refreshing chill.

5. Blend all the ingredients until smooth and creamy.

6. Taste the smoothie and adjust the consistency or sweetness by adding more liquid or fruit, if necessary.

7. Pour into a glass and enjoy your energizing green smoothie!

Note: Feel free to customize this recipe based on your preferences. You can add other greens like kale or Swiss chard, and you can experiment with different fruits or additional ingredients like ginger for an extra kick.

Golden Milk with Turmeric:

Ingredients:

- 2 cups of milk (dairy or plant-based like almond, coconut, or soy milk)

- 1 teaspoon ground turmeric

- 1/2 teaspoon ground cinnamon

- 1/4 teaspoon ground ginger

- A pinch of black pepper (enhances turmeric absorption)

- 1-2 teaspoons honey or maple syrup (adjust to taste)

- Optional: 1/2 teaspoon coconut oil for added richness

Instructions:

1. In a small saucepan, heat the milk over medium heat until it's warm but not boiling.

2. Add the turmeric, cinnamon, ginger, black pepper, and coconut oil (if using) to the warm milk.

3. Whisk the mixture continuously to ensure that the spices are well combined and there are no lumps.

4. Allow the mixture to simmer for about 5 minutes, stirring occasionally. Be careful not to let it boil.

5. Remove the saucepan from the heat and let it cool slightly.

6. Add honey or maple syrup to sweeten the golden milk, adjusting the amount to your liking. Stir well.

7. Strain the golden milk through a fine mesh sieve if you prefer a smoother texture, or you can enjoy it as is for a bit of texture.

8. Pour the golden milk into your favourite mug and savour this comforting and nutritious beverage.

Hydrating Infused Water:

1. **Citrus Mint Infusion**
    - **Ingredients:**
    - 1 lemon, thinly sliced
    - 1 lime, thinly sliced
    - Fresh mint leaves

- **Instructions:**
    1. Add lemon and lime slices to a pitcher.
    2. Toss in a handful of fresh mint leaves.
    3. Fill the pitcher with water and let it sit in the refrigerator for a few hours to allow the flavours to infuse.

2. **Berry Bliss Infusion**
    - **Ingredients:**
    - Mixed berries (strawberries, blueberries, raspberries)
    - 1 cucumber, thinly sliced

- **Instructions:**

1. Combine mixed berries and cucumber slices in a pitcher.

2. Fill the pitcher with water and refrigerate for a couple of hours.

3. **Cucumber Lemon Basil Refresher**

- **Ingredients:**

- 1 cucumber, thinly sliced

- 1 lemon, thinly sliced

- Fresh basil leaves

- **Instructions:**

1. Place cucumber and lemon slices in a pitcher.

2. Add fresh basil leaves.

3. Fill with water and let it infuse in the fridge for a refreshing taste.

4. **Tropical Pineapple Coconut Splash**

- **Ingredients:**

- Pineapple chunks

- Coconut water

- Fresh mint leaves (optional)

- **Instructions:**

1. Add pineapple chunks to a pitcher.

2. Pour coconut water over the pineapple.

3. Optionally, add a few fresh mint leaves for extra flavour.

4.   Refrigerate   and   allow   the   flavours   to   blend.

Conclusion

As you finish the **"Adrenal Fatigue Relief Diet Cookbook,"** I hope you've learned more than simply recipes. This cookbook is more than just a collection of recipes; it is a journey toward restoring your health. In the chapters, we've examined the fundamental relationship between mindful diet and adrenal health, equipping you with the knowledge to make choices that support your body and spirit.

Remember, this cookbook is not a fast fix, but rather a partner on your journey to long-term health. Accept the pleasure of cooking nutritious meals, savour the flavours that provide comfort, and savour the vigour with each attentive mouthful.

Amid the responsibilities and tensions of everyday life, may these recipes serve as a reminder to prioritize self-care. Your health is a valuable asset, and each meal is an opportunity to invest in it.

May you discover strength, balance, and resilience as you begin on this gastronomic journey. Here's to the tremendous tenacity of the human spirit, the healing power of food, and the joy of cooking.

Thank you for welcoming this cookbook into your home and life. May it serve as an inspiration, a source of sustenance, and a reminder that caring for oneself is a deep act of love.

64

Best wishes on your path to greater vigour and well-being.

Sincerely,

Vakare Rimkute